# Nourishment for a Healthy Life

**Joseph Anderson**

**Copyright © 2022**

# Table of content

# Introduction

In basic terms, the body has two altogether different and complex frameworks of fuel delivering sources. As energy is essential to the actual presence of human action and endurance, the two-energy style relies upon one another for help. This book shows you what food varieties give you the most energy.

It happens so habitually we resolve to happen with wellbeing and actual workout regime with zing and reasonably much ballyhoo as well; in any case, in the main seven-day stretch of going into the arrangement, all that subsides. Can anyone explain why we don't stay with the eating regimen designs, the early daytime running plans, and the actual activity designs that we make?

Also how may we guarantee we continue onward with these plans, for the good of our own and for the people that are subject to us?

Might it be said that you are eating just to fulfill your craving or to make your taste buds blissful? Or, then again, would you say you are eating to assume better control over your life? In this eBook, we perceive how you can make your life significantly more ideal basically by causing a guide that you toward eating accurately.

Energy is required for the different capabilities like upkeep of development, everyday exercises, practice and numerous developments or capabilities that are frequently underestimated. These are divided among the two energy frameworks.

In this day and age, only sometimes do any well-being and wellness plans work. What is the justification for their disturbing pace of disappointment? The world is significantly less restorative than it was twenty years prior. Much of this is credited to the changed food propensities for people.

# Chapter 1

# The Basics

The essential and first to be utilized energy framework is the high-impact framework. This framework involves oxygen for the capability of the muscles and requests a considerable amount from the general body framework.

This request for the most part expands the rate and profundity of breathing and blood supply, essentially given the relating increment of the pulse.

At the point when the body requires more energy, which can't be met because of the raised requirement for more oxygen, then the body framework consequently changed to the anaerobic energy framework. This framework can create energy without the need to utilize oxygen.

This energy is created through the appropriate or addressed utilization of food varieties. The food varieties devoured directly the kinds of energy levels everybody can create. Muscle weakness generally happens when all the energy sources are depleted, which can be credited to different reasons; the most convincing one relies particularly upon the sorts of food sources eaten.

There are a few classifications of food varieties that produce different helpful components for the human body framework, and taking note of the ones that make or improve the energy-creating sources is valuable to be aware of. Consequently, this information ought to assist the person with picking the right sorts of food sources.

The vigorous framework works by separating the starches, unsaturated fats, and amino acids in the food varieties devoured while the anaerobic framework sets energy free from the food varieties put away in the body, ordinarily during serious action sessions. If we find out about the disappointment of diets or rec center plans surrounding us regularly, it isn't their issue.

Generally, the issue of the people began with much upheaval about going through these plans, leaving out nothing for their associates and collaborators about it, and afterward didn't keep those projects. The people who forsake the activity or abstain from food midway don't see the benefits, normally and everyone faults the arrangement.

What the world necessities these days is certainly not a new well-being or workout regime or an eating routine. However, it requires inspiration. It needs the right kind of attitude to finish anything plan they have decided as far as possible.

If they can do that, the majority of the medical problems that are connected with the way of life circumstances will become outdated. What's more, we don't need to visit the sides of the earth to find this inspiration. The inspiration lies here, inside us; we have to look through it out and use it.

One age back, people wouldn't fantasize about getting anything that unhealthy food they might set up to take care of their countenances. These days, that's what we do so nonchalantly. "I'm eager" generally signifies "I need a burger or a wiener, possible with chips as an afterthought and some cola." And, "I'm on a careful nutritional plan" signifies "I'm on a synthetically ridden pill which will overcome my craving and deny my collection of nutrients." It's truly no big surprise that we are confronting so many medical problems today.

Our well-being is a mark of what we consume. The sorry condition that we're living in is not a singular issue  it's a worldwide issue. The world is eating mistakenly. Six in every ten people in the US are overweight, and the number will be eight in every ten people when we hit 2023.

Could it be said that we are genuinely pondering this? We aren't. Indeed, even as you're concentrating on this eBook, you probably have a parcel of chips as an afterthought. Do you have any idea that what you spent on that bundle, which is filling your stomach with the absolute most poisonous synthetics known to humankind, could rather have taken care of a thin young person in Ruanda?

However, it's not just about being magnanimous. It's about ourselves as well. Indeed, we must be self-centered. With such shocking well-being figures, would we confirm or deny that we are setting out toward destruction? We're certainly not eating right. Whatever overabundance stuff that brings - corpulence and the varying chronic sickness afterward - we must be ready for it.

So the following time, you see that a program has fizzled or is getting a great deal of analysis, recollect that the analysis isn't likely because the program remains in dangerous territory. As a rule, it is because individuals started with extraordinary expectations and afterward didn't follow the program as they ought to have.

The most vital thing that you want to keep your well-being and workout regime alive - much more pivotal than a teacher or a specialist - is your thought process. You are still up in the air to examine what is happening. In this way, you're overweight and are seeing pushing off a couple of pounds.

No rec center teacher from wherever on the planet will help you on the off chance that you don't go to sufficient lengths to have the right eating regimen and to adhere to your standard activity. Regardless of whether you're wiped out and are taking a gander at treatment, no doctor will help if not set in stone in following the treatment stage, whether it's taking the prescription at the right time or going without certain food sources.

# Chapter 2

# Your Mindset

We have wandered terribly with our dietary patterns hitherto. Assume control over won't improve, the first thing is mindfulness. We need to realize what food sources are right for us and what is not. We need to return to preparing and fathom what the supplements are that your body genuinely needs and in what sum.

Then we need to construct a dietary routine for ourselves as well as our friends and family, so we eat better. We need to eliminate every one of the food varieties that are unfavorable - the sugars, the fats, the starches. We don't genuinely need them - and consolidate food varieties that might support our wellbeing.

This sounds excessively long-winded, I get it. In any case, that is the main relief we have. On the off chance that we keep crunching on Oreos, we're never going to improve. In any case, there's trust. Trust lies in the way that there are a lot of food sources out there that are essentially basically as delectable as those horrendous unhealthy foods. However, we have barely any familiarity with them.

These are the food sources that we have barely any familiarity with yet, we probably could do without them or as we don't have the foggiest idea how to fix them, a sound cookbook might help you in figuring out grouped fascinating ways to solid cooking. Indeed, even with a similar kind of diet you eat, you can evoke a few truly heavenly sound dishes. Indeed, it's all a lot conceivable. You can change your dietary patterns to a major degree, while simultaneously taking care of your sense of taste.

The truth of the matter is that the weight reduction industry is mindful in a critical manner of this defeat of the created human race.

They show us glamorous before-after photos of an individual with a foot-long sub and afterward the very fellow with 6-pack abs and let us know that the eating routine made that conceivable. Nonetheless, the truth of the matter is, if we somehow managed to get our head together, we may effectively do that as well, without burning through 1000s of dollars on those eating regimens. Furthermore, what do we need to do?

Control what we consume, Enjoy the actual effort. Presently, is that a lot to achieve? Don't we owe that to our body that has served us so well for such an extremely long time? Don't we owe that to ourselves and our friends and family?

Throughout the long term, honey has been demonstrated to be the one supporting power behind the energy circle. Helping the human body in different regions is preeminent and still unparalleled in its energy-creating element. Honey is nature's most regular energy promoter. It likewise goes about as a viable invulnerability framework developer while giving the regular solution to a large group of different illnesses as well.

Energy is vital to the smooth streaming normal of a routine pattern of any individual. Along these lines, finding energy sources that are both reliable and sound are essential to staying in shape and cheerful.

# Chapter 3

# A Good Pair

The regular advantages of honey have been broadly recognized and acknowledged. Other than its incredible taste, honey is likewise a characteristic wellspring of carbs, which is an energy creator for supporting execution, perseverance, and diminishing degrees of muscle weakness.

This is particularly valuable for competitors. The sugar content in the honey assists with assuming a part in forestalling exhaustion during exercise meetings and instructional courses for a sports fan.

These sugar make-ups are partitioned into glucose and fructose and capabilities in various, however, commending ways.

The glucose content in the honey is by and large consumed at a quicker rate and radiates a prompt jolt of energy while the fructose works at a more slow speed for a more maintainable and delayed energy payment. With regards to tending to glucose levels in the body framework, honey has been known to assist with keeping the levels consistent.

As honey is a charming food item and it's normal in its structure, devouring its anything but truly challenging activity. Individuals of any age are by and large, very ready to consume honey in any of it going structures. It's even well known with kids.

The energy delivered from consuming a modest quantity of honey day-to-day assists kids with adapting to the actual types of everyday school exercises and sports responsibilities.

For the grown-ups, too consuming a day-to-day little portion of honey can go far in keeping the energy levels at their best during a requesting day at work. Making sandwiches with honey went with different fillings is one approach to making a wonderful tidbit.

Applying honey on a newly toasted cut of bread is likewise a welcome breakfast elective. Adding honey to drinks as opposed to utilizing sugar is energized. The vast majority today need a handy solution for their energy-supporting requirements and this typically comes in the undesirable types of sports beverages, espresso, and refined carbs like sugar and keeping in mind that bread.

However, these produce the ideal elevated energy levels. It ought to be noticed that this energy is genuinely brief and the sleepiness that follows is generally more intensely felt. Thusly picking to consume some type of entire grains isn't just a superior other option but at the same time is a lot better.

Entire grains give the energy that arrives in a more perplexing structure that separates over a more extended timeframe. This then makes the stage for supporting the energy levels for longer periods.

On account of its more complicated make up, the entire grains accompany a variety of helpful components like minerals, nutrients, phytonutrient and fiber which are additionally wealthy in fiber. Adding the entire grain fixings in any dish frequently finishes the flavor or upgrades it through and through. Entire grains can be the different structures like wheat, oat, grain, maize, earthy colored rice, faro, spelled, emmer, einkorn, rye, millet, buckwheat and some more.

These can then be made into different items like entire wheat flour, entire wheat bread, entire wheat pasta, moved oats or oat groats, triticale flour, popcorn and teff flour.

The advantages of consuming entire grains reliably can assist with diminishing the gamble of coronary illness, lower cholesterol levels safeguard against many kinds of malignant growth, and aid weight the board. Entire grains ought not to be mistaken for their lesser and more refined "cousin". However, refined grains have a few advantages, it is in every case better to decide overall grain choices.

Nuts are a significant wellspring of supplements for both human and creature utilization. Being wealthy in an entire host of essential supplements, it very well may be eaten in its crude structure, cooked or as an added substance to currently previous dishes. Though nuts are characterized as a hard-shelled natural product, numerous food varieties are remembered for the nut family.

Various sorts of meats, for the most part, add two different flavors, but the best kind is the one with however much lean meat content as could be expected. Its undisputed truth is that the meats that contain a lot of fat are a culinary treat for sure. However  for well-being purposes finding the opportunity to comprehend the advantages of consuming lean meats is exceptionally very shrewd.

# Chapter 4

# Great Proteins And Oils

It is presently considered normal information that nuts significantly help to hold a ton of illnesses within proper limits or from happening by any means.

For example, nuts have been known to have the option to keep the chance of coronary heart illnesses showing in any event for those entire come from a long queue of relatives with this issue.

Consuming nuts like almonds and pecans has been known to bring down serum cholesterol fixations on the body framework. Nuts are additionally energetically suggested for those people experiencing insulin obstruction issues like diabetics.

Going to nuts rather than unhealthy food to suppress desires is likewise another better other option. Containing fundamental unsaturated fats is likewise one more in addition to the moment that it comes to picking nuts as a better other option. Since nuts are sound and can be consumed in their crude structure, it is additionally one more added benefit to keeping these around and convenient as bites.

Almonds are frequently used to standardize blood lipids as a result of their gradual process qualities, which help to keep the glucose levels reliably sound. Rich in a changed measure of various supplements, the almond is a well-known added substance to the flat eating regimen of most Mediterranean individuals.

The Brazil nut is likewise another nutritious nut that accompanies its arrangement of advantages when consumed with some restraint. Noted for its omega-3 unsaturated fat substance, the Brazil nut is likewise a decent wellspring of calcium.

Cashew nut is one more extremely famous nut that is many times consumed as a salted bite. Anyway, it would be a lot better food item without the expansion of salt, as it is as of now a seriously tasty nut all alone. In certain regions of the planet these nuts are made into oils.

The choice cycle ought to be finished with a touch of information as relying exclusively upon what the unaided eye sees isn't sufficient. By and large lean meats got from hamburger, cuts ought to incorporate round, hurl, sirloin and tenderloin while the cuts of pork or sheep would comprise tenderloin, flank hacks, and leg. The least fatty pieces of the poultry would be the bosom region without the skin.

However  there are many reasons individuals wipe out meat from their everyday eating regimen. There is no proof to show that this is a positive or negative decision, nor would it be a good idea for it to be trailed by all.

Anyway the significant highlight note here is the decision of the kinds of meats that would make the utilization sound and this would commonly mean meats with a lesser measure of fat substance. However, white meat is in no way, shape, or form ailing in fat substance. It is by examination substantially less in fat substance than red meats. The healthy benefit of consuming lean meats is very broad and adjusted.

Lean meats have a by and large higher and cleaner content of protein, which is a vital contributing element to the central underlying and useful advancement of every cell food and development.

Lean meats are likewise a decent wellspring of fundamental amino acids, especially sulfur amino acids. When contrasted with the stomach-related rates, the proteins in meats work quicker than the ones contained in the beans and entire wheat range.

Lean meat is likewise a decent wellspring of iron. Since lack of iron is moderate, it is frequently not identified until a later stage when pallor has been created.

Here is all the rationale you'd expect to keep practicing good eating habits. How about we promptly dive into the subject?

# Chapter 5

# Benefits

You Get Healthier :-  We could have entire assortment of books about the well-being benefits of eating accurately despite everything, it wouldn't exactly cover what benefits truly exist. The main benefit is that you gain control over your weight.

By eating accurately  you similarly verify that your metabolic capabilities - most remarkably  your resistant framework and your gastrointestinal framework  continue to work accurately. You're in like manner shielded from arranged ongoing illnesses right from cardiovascular sicknesses like coronary course sickness and hypertension to diabetes.

## More Cost Effective

Practicing good eating habits implies you spend significantly less. Your bills at the stores descend radically and you don't dive farther into charge card obligation assuming that is as of now an issue with you. Likewise, you save an immense pack on all the medical services costs you'd require if any issue surfaces in light of your food gorging propensities.

## Fewer Toxins In Your Body

A lot of food varieties these days are harmful due to the engineered synthetic compounds present in them. While you're endeavoring to eat accurately, you are significantly less prone to get these poisons into your body as one of the fundamental doctrines of eating accurately is that you shouldn't eat anything that is manmade.

Furthermore, if you eat less, you'll similarly have the option to diminish indecencies like smoking and liquor addiction. A glass of lager is practically inseparable from a night out with the young men. If you eat less, you won't need the larger too. Additionally, you won't need that (at least one) required smoke that you will more often than not have after every dinner.

## More Physical Lifestyle

At the point when you eat better, you'll observe that you can take care of your responsibilities in a greatly improved manner. You can practice more  travel more, play more, work more and in this manner make your life more useful.

That beats being a fat lazy pig and relaxing around on the sofa the entire day right? You can likewise be more engaged with your companions and friends and family and that advances your life.

## Great Social Life

Disregard fat fetishism, People who are overweight don't look engaging. There are serious areas of strength for an untouchable weight on some unacceptable spots of the body. On the off chance that you're attempting to find an accomplice, your fat may in a real sense disrupt the general flow. Not just that  people who have zero control over their dietary patterns and thus their weight are peered downward on by society as being people who have zero control over their essential desires.

This kind of brain research exists however not very many people will talk about it. At the point when you eat accurately, you'll find that such issues vanish.

There are a ton of well-known eats less available these days  however  the greater part of them are unfortunate and periodically even risky. This will clarify how to eat a solid, adjusted diet forever and avoid undesirable weight control plans.

# Chapter 6

## Find out the number of calories your body is expected to work with consistently

This number might differ fiercely, contingent upon your digestion and how dynamic you are. On the off chance that you're the kind of person who lies on ten hammers out plainly smelling a cut of pizza, then your consistently caloric admission should remain roughly 2000 calories for men, and 1500 calories for ladies.

Your weight similarly has an impact in that: More calories are proper for normally greater people and fewer calories for smaller people. If you're the kind of person who can eat without acquiring a pound, or you're genuinely dynamic, you could wish to build your everyday caloric admission by 1000-2000 calories, a piece less for ladies.

### Try not to fear greasy food sources

You need to devour fat from food varieties for your body to accurately run. However, selecting the right kinds of fats: Most creature fats and a couple of vegetable oils are high

in the kind of fats that raise your LDL cholesterol levels;
the foul cholesterol is significant.

Not the same as mainstream thinking, gobbling cholesterol
doesn't unavoidably raise how much cholesterol is in your
body. Assuming you give your body the right apparatuses,
it will flush additional cholesterol from your body. Those
instruments are monounsaturated unsaturated fats, which
you should attempt to consistently consume. Food
varieties that are wealthy in monounsaturated
unsaturated fats are olive oil, nuts, fish oil, and grouped
seed oils.

## Eat a lot of the right carbs

You need to eat food varieties high in carbs since they're
your body's central wellspring of energy. Try to select the
right carbs. Straightforward carbs like sugar and refined
flour are immediately consumed by the body's
gastrointestinal framework.

This prompts a kind of carb over-burden, and your body
discharges immense measures of insulin to fight the
over-burden. Not exclusively is the abundance of insulin
awful on your heart, but it empowers weight gain.

Eat a lot of carbs, yet consume carbs that are gradually processed by the body, for example, entire grain flour, veggies, oats, and natural grains.

## Eat greater dinners from the get-go in the day

Your digestion decelerates around the finish of the night and is less proficient at processing food varieties. That implies a greater amount of the power put away in the food will be stacked away as fat and your body will not retain as numerous supplements from the dinner.

Have a go at eating a medium-sized feast for breakfast, a major dinner for lunch, and a little dinner for supper. Even better, endeavor to consume 4-6 little feasts over the run of your day.

## Give yourself a cheat dinner

Cheating doesn't mean glutting on every one of some unacceptable food varieties one time each week; it infers partaking in the food you genuinely love one time each week.

Two or three cuts of pizza on Sundays, or a colossal cut of twofold chocolate cake on Saturdays.

This cheat feast will assist you with staying with the adjustment of diet, and in a couple of ways, it's truly great for your body. Exceptional events, similar to birthday events in the family, consider cheat dinners.

## Get the propensity for eating gradually

It will fulfill you with fewer calories and will thwart indulging and corpulence with every one of its ramifications.

## Drink a lot of water

It causes you to feel more conscious and stimulated, does ponder for your skin, and causes you to feel more full so you end up eating less! Chopping down pop and supplanting it with water will do ponders for you.